Health Care Policy and Politics

Health Care Policy and Politics

Lessons from Four Countries

Edited by Robert B. Helms

The AEI Press

Publisher for the American Enterprise Institute
WASHINGTON, D.C.

1993

Library of Congress Cataloging-in-Publication Data

Health care policy and politics : lessons from four countries /
    edited by Robert B. Helms.
        p.   cm.
    Includes bibliographical references.
    ISBN 0-8447-3838-7
    1. Medical policy.   2. Health planning.
I. Helms, Robert B.
RA393.H413   1993
362.1—dc20   93-29700
                                                        CIP

1 2 3 4 5 6 7 8 9 10

THE AEI PRESS
Publisher for the American Enterprise Institute
1150 Seventeenth Street, N.W.
Washington, D.C. 20036

Printed in the United States of America

NWST
IAEA6110

Contents

Contributors

ROBERT B. HELMS is a resident scholar and director of health policy studies at the American Enterprise Institute. He has written and lectured extensively on health policy, health economics, and pharmaceutical economic issues. He is the editor of AEI's recent publication on health policy, *American Health Policy: Critical Issues for Reform.* From 1981 to 1989, Dr. Helms served as assistant secretary for planning and evaluation and deputy assistant secretary for health policy in the Department of Health and Human Services.

WARREN GREENBERG is professor of health economics and health care sciences and a senior fellow at the Center for Health Policy Research at George Washington University. He is an authority on the subjects of competition and regulation in health care. He has written numerous articles on the economics of health care and has edited or written nine books. Dr. Greenberg continues his research on the Israeli and Dutch health care systems, as well as information dissemination, antitrust, competition, regulation, and rationing in the U.S. health care sector. Dr. Greenberg's newest book is *Competition, Regulation, and Rationing.*

ALAN MAYNARD is professor of economics and director of the Centre for Health Economics at the University of York, England. He has taught in New Zealand, Italy, and Sweden. He has worked as a consultant for the European Commission, the World Health Organization, and the World Bank. His interest in health care reform led to the production of *Public-Private Mix for Health*, coedited with Gordon McLachlan, and involvement in the NHS health care reform of the Thatcher government.

EDWARD NEUSCHLER is director of the Department of Policy Development and Research for the Health Insurance Association of America. His department provides analytical and research support for the association's policy development process, dealing with a wide variety of issues facing HIAA on the national level. Mr. Neuschler was closely involved in developing HIAA's proposals for expanding Medicaid to cover all the poor and has also assisted HIAA's long-term care staff in developing the public program portion of HIAA's strategy for financing long-term care in the United States. He has significant experience in managed health care with a Medicaid focus, health care cost-containment approaches, and government-financed long-term care. Among his many publications is *Canadian Health Care: The Implications of Public Health Insurance*.

SEAN SULLIVAN is president of the National Business Coalition Forum on Health. The forum leads a growing movement of employer coalitions in more than sixty cities to get better quality health care for their workers, while holding down costs. Mr. Sullivan works with the Jackson Hole Group on the design of managed competition and informs members of the Conservative Democratic Forum as well as Republican leaders about community-based reforms being made. His previous work has examined the causes of rising health care costs and the development of private and public strategies for managing the cost and quality of care. Before joining the NBCFH, he was executive vice president of New Directions for Policy, where he completed a study of the German health care system. He has also served as assistant director of the Council on Wage and Price Stability and as a scholar at the American Enterprise Institute.

Health Care Policy and Politics

ONE

Introduction

Robert B. Helms

The American people face important decisions in this field at a time when it is still difficult to obtain the information on which such a decision should be based. This is true not only for the layman, but also for the professional student of society who can devote much time to such a task. He finds it far from easy to form an adequate picture of what has been learned by the experiments with state medicine in other countries.

FRIEDRICH A. HAYEK
Preface, Financing Medical Care:
An Appraisal of Foreign Programs

The frustration expressed by Friedrich Hayek thirty years ago continues today. As dissatisfaction about the performance of the U.S. health care system

---

I am indebted to my friend and colleague W. Allen Wallis for bringing to my attention Friedrich Hayek's preface to *Financing Medical Care: An Appraisal of Foreign Programs*, edited by Helmut Shoeck (Caldwell, Idaho: Caxton Printers, 1962), pp. v–viii. Hayek's preface was reprinted in *The American Enterprise*, vol. 3, no. 3 (May/June 1992), p. 16.

grows, increasing attention has been given to how health care is delivered and financed in other countries. But as Hayek warns, learning health policy lessons from the experiences of other countries is far from easy. The task is complicated by, in slightly more contemporary terminology, a lack of data and good analysis.

Without presuming that we can overcome these difficulties, this volume presents both data and good analysis about health care policies in four countries: Canada, Germany, the Netherlands, and the United Kingdom. The lessons for the United States, however, will be more in keeping with Hayek's frustration and his implied warning to be careful about what we learn. Each author has been asked to present information about the performance of one country's health care system and to analyze how politics have affected its performance. Our objective is to question the simplistic way in which we in the United States have often been asked to emulate the health policies of other countries.

A relatively large body of literature on international comparisons of health care systems and policies is emerging.[1] While many countries have features of interest to the U.S. debate, this volume concentrates on the four countries that are most often held up as examples. Each author has extensive experience in

---

1. For a sample of this literature, each containing numerous other references, see *Health Care Financing Review, 1989 Annual Supplement,* Health Care Financing Administration, vol. 11, no. 1 (Fall 1989); *Health Affairs,* vol. 10, no. 3 (Fall 1991) and vol. 11, no. 1 (Spring 1992); and Laurene A. Graig, *Health of Nations: An International Perspective on U.S. Health Care Reform* (Washington, D.C.: Wyatt Company, 1991). For a discussion of future research on international comparisons, see Kathleen N. Lohr, Karl Yordy, Polly F. Harrison, and Annetine C. Gelijns, "Health Care Systems: Lessons from International Comparisons," *Health Affairs,* vol. 11, no. 4 (Winter 1992), pp. 239–41.

the analysis of health care policy issues and has recently completed research relating to that country. Each author was instructed to minimize descriptive material and to concentrate on how the country's health care system is functioning and how it is being affected by political forces. Instead of looking at stylized models, these articles examine how each system has been affected by real world forces such as demographic changes, the power of special interests, and politics. This interest in political effects is not misplaced. If anything about the future of U.S. health policy can be easily predicted, it is that it will continue to be a central issue in federal and state politics.

Basic Health Care Data in OECD Countries

As background, this introduction presents some basic data comparing various features of health care in the United States and the other four countries covered in the volume. The Organization for Economic Cooperation and Development has published extensive data on health care for its twenty-four member-countries.[2] Figures 1–1 through 1–3 present basic data about health care expenditures in the United States and the four countries featured in this volume. Figure 1–1 presents the most used statistic in international comparisons, total health expenditures as a percentage of the gross domestic product. This figure indicates the importance of the health care sector in the total economy of each country.

---

2. See Jean-Pierre Poullier, "Health Data File: Overview and Methodology," *Health Care Financing Review*, pp. 111–94. Except where otherwise noted, the data presented in these figures are taken from the Organization for Economic Cooperation and Development software package, *The OECD Health Data Program*, English version 1.05, 1993.

FIGURE 1–1
Total Health Expenditures as a Percentage of Gross Domestic Product in Five Nations, 1980 and 1991

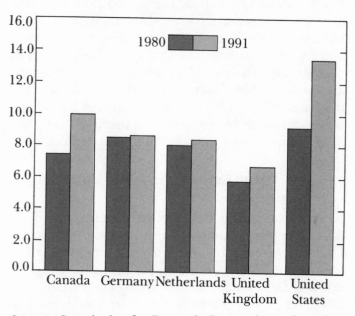

SOURCE: Organization for Economic Cooperation and Development, *The OECD Health Data Program,* software package, English version, 1.05, 1993.

The United States had the highest absolute level of expenditures in both 1980 and 1990 and the highest rate of increase of the five countries.

Figure 1–2 shows the relationship between per capita GDP and per capita health expenditures for all twenty-four OECD countries, as presented by George J. Schieber and Jean-Pierre Poullier.[3] As they point

---

3. Schieber and Poullier, "International Health Care Expenditure Trends, 1987," *Health Affairs,* vol. 8, no. 3 (Fall 1989), p. 173.

FIGURE 1–2
PER CAPITA HEALTH EXPENDITURES AND PER CAPITA
GROSS DOMESTIC PRODUCT FOR OECD COUNTRIES,
1991

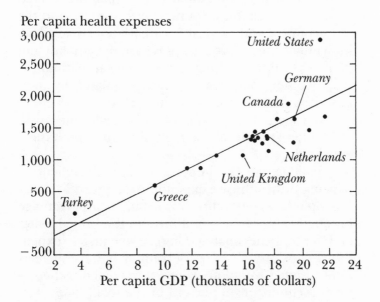

SOURCE: Adapted from George J. Schieber, Jean-Pierre Poullier, and Leslie Greenwald, "Health Spending, Delivery and Outcomes in OECD Countries," *Health Affairs* (Summer 1993).

out, "Expenditures in the United States ($2,051) were more than double the OECD average ($934) and 38 percent higher than expenditures in Canada ($1,483), the second highest country."[4] While the United States is clearly above the trend line, there are two basic interpretations of why the United States is

4. Schieber and Poullier, "Overview of International Comparisons of Health Care Expenditures," *Health Care Financing Review*, Fall 1989, p. 4 and table 3.

an outlier in such a comparison. The first, and most common, is that this is evidence of the waste and inefficiency inherent in our system of open-ended government payment and private health insurance. A second interpretation, however, is that the United States is the wealthiest country in this group and the only country with a health care system that allows individuals the freedom to purchase the amount and kind of health care they desire. The implication is that if other countries were less regulated by their governments, the individuals in those countries might spend a higher proportion of their wealth on health care. There may be an element of truth in both these explanations.

To illustrate the importance of government financing of health care expenditures, figure 1–3 presents public expenditures on health as a percentage of total health care expenditures in the United States and the countries analyzed here. Some private expenditures are present in every country but are smallest in the United Kingdom, where government expenditures account for 83 percent of the total. (Sweden is the highest among OECD countries at about 90 percent.) The United States, where most employed people are covered by private insurance, has the lowest proportion of government payment.[5]

Figure 1–4 illustrates demographic projections of the increasing proportion of aged people relative

---

5. But C. Eugene Steuerle points out that if the value of tax revenues (tax expenditures) lost because of the exclusion of the value of employer-provided health insurance and other hidden costs are counted, the U.S. government's role would be approximately 51 percent. Steuerle, "The Search for Adaptable Health Policy through Financed-Based Reform," in Robert B. Helms, ed., *American Health Policy: Critical Issues for Reform* (Washington, D.C.: AEI Press, 1993), p. 335, and figure 14–1.

FIGURE 1–3
PUBLIC HEALTH EXPENDITURES AS A PERCENTAGE OF TOTAL HEALTH EXPENDITURES IN FIVE COUNTRIES, 1991

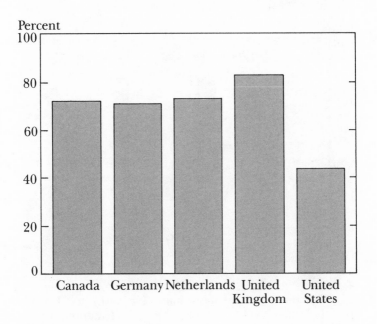

SOURCE: Organization for Economic Cooperation and Development, *The OECD Health Data Program,* software package, English version 1.05, 1993.

to the working-age populations. This trend is a growing problem for almost all countries, especially for the developed nations with government health programs for the aged that are paid for by taxes on the working population. The basic choice of cutting future benefits or raising taxes to meet these obligations is a common topic in health policy discussions in almost all countries, especially in the United States

FIGURE 1–4
The Aged Population Relative to the Working-Age Population for Selected Countries, 1980 and 2020

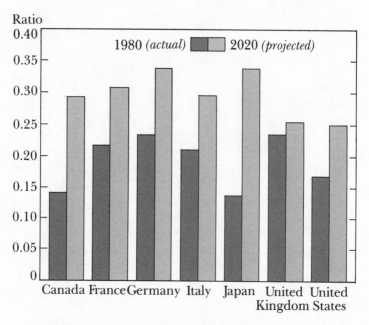

NOTE: Aged population = those aged sixty-five and over; working age population = those aged fifteen to sixty-four.
SOURCE: Organization for Economic Cooperation and Development, *Aging Populations: The Social Policy Implications* (Paris: OECD, 1988), table 14, p. 32.

and the four countries covered in this volume. The increasing competitiveness of world markets and worker resistance to new taxes are putting added pressure on governments to improve the efficiency and cost-effectiveness of health care.

The Basic Issues

Many other comparisons could be made among these five countries, but these four should serve to introduce the basic issues that are driving the debate about health policy: costs, access, and financial stability. Principally, people look to policies in other countries for lessons about improving the efficiency of health care delivery. The concept of efficiency combines both satisfying consumer preferences (delivering the kind of health care people want) and producing the desired amount with the least sacrifice of valuable resources. Policy discussions about almost any kind of product or service question the ability of private markets to achieve efficiency and the loss of economic efficiency that people are willing to sacrifice for the political benefit of some subset of society. Nowhere is this debate more complicated than in health care: many feel that the principles of market efficiency cannot be made to work in this service area. Experiences of other governments that have adopted policies to control expenditures take on added importance for those who hold this view. They point to the record in foreign countries of lower absolute levels of health expenditures and lower rates of growth as evidence that such direct government intervention can control health expenditures in the United States.

Although this characterization of the health policy reform debate is oversimplified, it illustrates that the debate hinges on two questions of efficacy: the efficacy of market-based policies and the efficacy of government expenditure controls. In a market-based health care system, can consumers get information to make informed decisions about health care matters?

Do prices give the correct signals for efficiency, or are they biased by insurance and monopoly power? Conversely, in countries with more government controls, has health care been delivered in a way that reduces real waste (and real costs) to consumers? Or has the objective of controls been subverted to the advantage of special interests at the expense of consumers? Or as some public choice and economic theories of regulations imply,[6] has the substitution of government controls for market incentives worked to the advantage of politicians and politically strong interest groups at the expense of both consumers and producers?

The authors of these essays were not asked to answer these questions or to determine the best health policies for the United States. But their analysis of the policies and politics in each country should give new meaning to Hayek's thirty-year-old warning that it is difficult to learn from other countries. Perhaps the central theme of these essays is that each country has based its health policy on its unique set of economic conditions and political preferences. If it is now time for the United States to reform its health care system, we too must devise a unique set of policies.

---

6. See, for example, Mark Pauly, "Why Is Health Care So Hard to Reform?" in Robert B. Helms, ed., *American Health Policy: Critical Issues for Reform* (Washington, D.C.: AEI Press, 1993), pp. 317–33; Sam Peltzman, "Toward a More General Theory of Regulation," *Journal of Law and Economics*, vol. 19 (1976), pp. 221–40.

nance imaging machines or computerized tomography scanners; all major surgery and high-technology diagnostic tests are done in hospitals. Canada's bed-to-population ratio is higher than ours. Hospitals admission rates are similar, but the average length of stay is 50 percent longer there, and occupancy rates are higher.[3]

How Canada Pays Providers. Hospitals negotiate their total operating budgets with the provincial health plans and are paid directly in a lump sum, not patient-by-patient. Thus, there is no billing for covered hospital care. Capital improvements, handled separately, must be approved in advance by the province. In most provinces, there is no allowance for depreciation. Even when capital improvements are funded entirely by local government or private philanthropy, the associated operating costs are still part of the total budget and must be approved by the province. This results in centralized government control over the supply of hospital services.

For physicians, provinces periodically negotiate fee increases with provincial medical associations. Physicians are paid on a fee-for-service basis according to the approved fee schedule. The provincial health plans are the sole payers for physicians' services. Physicians must accept the provincial plan's payment as payment in full; no balance billing of patients is permitted—a fairly recent change.[4] As a result, physician fees in Canada have escalated much less rapidly than in the United States. The increase from 1971 to 1985 in the fees of U.S. physicians exceeded

---

3. Ibid., pp. 18–19.
4. That is, physicians are not permitted to charge patients amounts that exceed the provincial plan's payment.

general inflation by 22.3 percent, while fees of Canadian physicians fell 18 percent behind inflation.[5]

But fee controls tend to motivate physicians to provide more services (or to bill separately for services previously packaged together) to maintain income. Canada's physicians apparently did just that. Between 1971 and 1985, per capita utilization of physicians' services grew much more rapidly in Canada: 67.8 percent, compared with 49.4 percent in the United States.[6]

In response, provinces have tried various methods to control the growth of total spending on physicians' services. Several have reduced fee increases to account for greater-than-expected increases in utilization. Quebec implemented an income limit for individual physicians in the mid-1970s, and Ontario has recently followed suit.

Use of nurse practitioners and physicians' assistants is more limited in Canada than in the United States. And there is virtually no American-style managed care. Ontario and Quebec do have community health centers that operate on global budgets. Ontario's are mostly in underserved areas; Quebec's are available in almost all communities. Ontario also has some physician groups called health services organizations that are paid on a per capita basis. The capitation payment covers all physician services provided by the HSO, but the HSO is not at risk for hospital care. Because of the global budgeting system, there is no way to calculate the hospital costs incurred by particular patients. The HSO does receive incen-

5. Morris L. Barer, Robert G. Evans, and Roberta J. Labelle, "Fee Controls as Cost Control: Tales from the Frozen North," *Milbank Quarterly*, vol. 66, no. 1 (1988), table A3, p. 51.
6. Ibid.

tive payments if its patients use hospital care less often than expected.

Both Ontario and Quebec have been talking about establishing entities that would look more like American health maintenance organizations. But nothing of this sort is yet operational.

The Canadian Record on Cost Containment and Access

With respect to cost containment, Canada has been successful in controlling health spending as a percentage of total economic output (figure 2–1), although its spending is the second highest in the developed world. If we look at the growth of per capita spending over time, we get a somewhat different picture. Figure 2–2 shows how per capita spending has grown in Canada and the United States relative to spending in 1960.[7] The similarity in growth trends is striking. There is some evidence that the growth rate in Canada has slowed since 1986, but the Canadian figures after 1987 are preliminary, not final, and are subject to revision.

We get the same general impression from figure 2–3, which shows Canadian health spending per capita as a percentage of U.S. health spending per capita over time. In per capita terms, Canada spends three quarters or less of what the United States spends. But Canada is solidly in second place among the developed nations for per capita spending. The stability of the percentage up until the past few years, moreover, is quite striking: Canada was spending considerably

---

7. In the computation of growth rates shown in figure 2–2, growth due to general inflation, as measured by the implicit price deflator for GDP in each country, has been omitted.

FIGURE 2–1
Total National Health Expenditures as a Percentage of Gross Domestic Product in Canada and the United States, 1960–1991

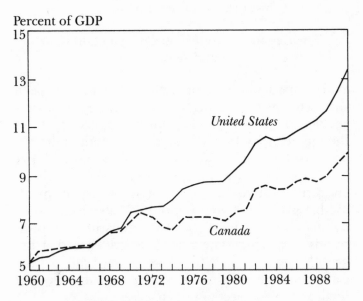

Percent of GDP

Source: Organization for Economic Cooperation and Development, *The OECD Health Data Program,* software package, English version 1.05, 1993.

less than the United States well before its public health insurance system was implemented.

Thus, while Canada has apparently done somewhat better than we have in controlling health cost escalation, clearly there was no dramatic change in the growth trend when Canada implemented universal public insurance. According to this experience, we should not expect public health insurance to be a

FIGURE 2–2
Cumulative Increase in Real Health Spending
per Capita for Canada and the United States,
1960–1991

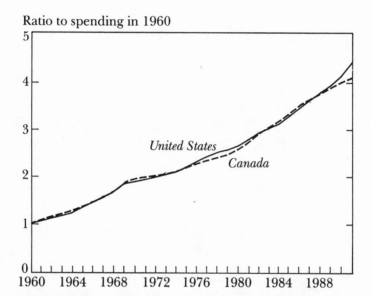

Ratio to spending in 1960

SOURCE: Organization for Economic Cooperation and Development, *The OECD Health Data Program,* software package, English version 1.05, 1993.

silver bullet, a simple, magical solution to our health care cost problems.

Clearly, Canadians enjoy excellent access to primary and ambulatory care. There are no bills or paperwork anywhere in the system. No one worries about financial catastrophe due to medical bills. Even physicians, though they may carp about the fee limits, feel better off than their southern neighbors, because

17

FIGURE 2–3
CANADIAN HEALTH CARE SPENDING PER CAPITA AS A PERCENTAGE OF U.S. HEALTH CARE SPENDING PER CAPITA, 1960–1991

Percent of U.S. spending per capita

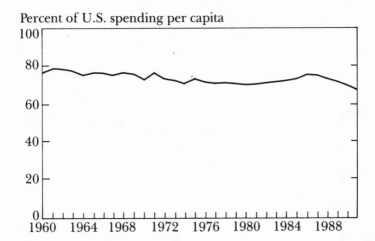

SOURCE: Organization for Economic Cooperation and Development, *The OECD Health Data Program,* software package, English version 1.05, 1993.

no one second-guesses their treatment recommendations. Canadians love their medicare system.

But the cost of maintaining free and unconstrained access to primary care is significant restrictions on the supply of expensive high-tech services. The United States, for example, has eight times as many magnetic resonance imaging scanners per capita as Canada and six times as many lithotripters.[8]

---

8. Dale A. Rublee, "Medical Technology in Canada, Germany,

Long waiting lists are routinely reported in the Canadian press for many medical procedures and technology introduced in the 1980s: coronary artery bypass grafts, hip replacements, lithotripsy, cataract removal with lens implant, MRI scans. Probably most real emergencies go to the head of the queue, but clearly many people suffer a reduced quality of life and heightened anxiety while they wait for needed treatment.

In the past few years, Canada's severe budget problems—the accumulated debt is worse than America's as a percentage of total national output—have led the federal government to freeze its contribution to the provincial health plans. That, combined with the recession, has sorely squeezed provincial budgets and limited the funds available for health care. In the past year or so, the papers have been full of stories about hospitals closing beds and laying off staff because of budget constraints.

There is no need to dwell on this—the stories have been widely reported in the press. The lesson to be drawn is that rationing by queue is the inevitable result of government attempts to control costs by restricting health care budgets while publicly espousing a commitment to universal access. Because anything new represents an additional cost, bureaucratic budget control discourages innovation, perpetuates existing inefficiencies, and leads to creeping obsolescence.

Lessons for the United States

What can the United States learn from Canada? The way government cost control operates is clear from

----

and the United States," *Health Affairs*, vol. 8, no. 3 (Fall 1989), pp. 178–81.

the Canadian experience. A budget is a blunt instrument. It cannot find and excise the unnecessary care—low-tech as well as high-tech—that we all know is the real fat and waste in the system. Further, because it is politically difficult to stop paying for services that have been covered or to restrict access to them, the easy way out for the budgeteer is just to say no to anything new.

Given our vast overcapacity in health care, the United States would not run into waiting lists per se anytime soon if we went to a single government health plan. This did not become a significant problem in Canada until perhaps fifteen years after public health insurance was introduced.

The effect in the United States would be subtler and more insidious. Development of new technology would slow significantly, simply because of the risk that the single government plan would decide not to pay for the new technology. No one would be willing to make the upfront investment needed to develop technology.

In the political arena, there are significant differences between Canada and the United States, factors that make it easier to attain consensus on major societal issues in Canada. First, Canadians in general have a more benevolent view of government as the means by which people do things collectively. Second, Canada's parliamentary system makes it easier to take positive action once a majority has decided which approach it prefers.

Even with these cultural and political differences, the current Canadian system was not adopted overnight. It grew gradually, step by step, over a period of more than forty years. Universal coverage of hospital care came first, beginning in the late 1940s in

Saskatchewan and British Columbia, with federal legislation following in 1955 and all provinces on board by 1960. Public coverage of physicians' services came later, after a debate which sounds familiar to American ears. Again, Saskatchewan led the way in 1962. Subsequent federal legislation in 1966 led all provinces to implement universal public plans for medical services between 1968 and 1971. Finally, balance billing and user charges were not specifically outlawed until 1984.[9] Moreover, the development of public health insurance in Canada began and was largely completed when the organization of health care services was much less complicated than now.

The United States should follow a course that encourages continued development and growth of managed care for cost containment, combined with public subsidies and insurance reform to make private health insurance available to those who cannot now afford it. Adopting a government-run public insurance scheme like Canada's would dull the cutting edge of medical progress and leave us with "hurry up and wait" health care. We can do better.

9. Neuschler, *Canadian Health Care*, pp. 9–14.

21

THREE

An American Perspective on the German Health Care System

Sean Sullivan

Politicians in the nation's capital have had a continuing infatuation with the health care systems of other industrialized countries (except South Africa). But their attention span is short and their affections inconstant, keeping us all wondering where they will look next for *the* model that the United States should adopt. Indeed, there is a "system of the session" fashion on Capitol Hill, just as various versions of industrial policy are donned and then discarded like Parisian garments. Observers of Washington styles agree that Canada and Germany are the centers of *haute couture* in health policy.

Germany's inclusion here may seem surprising to many Americans, who assume that our next-door neighbors to the north must be much like us and, therefore, that a health care system that apparently pleases most of them would suit us as well. With apologies to Quebec, though, Canada—or at least Ontario, its heart—remains a bastion of British cus-

tom and outlook. While most Americans retain a
fondness for Britain, this does not extend to its health
care system. On closer inspection, we find that the
Canadian system is a first cousin of the British and
would not be accepted if adopted here.

Turning away from Canada after their earlier
dalliance, then, more lawmakers are finding Germany
alluring—at least from a distance. Its health care
system looks much more like ours, with a large role
for insurers and employers and more choice for individuals. And it has been far more successful than
the United States or Canada at containing the growth
of spending. But a longer look is necessary to find
out if this, too, is just another infatuation that will
fade on closer acquaintance.

History and Philosophy

Germany's health care system is difficult to classify in
terms of the degree of government involvement. Unlike Canada's, it is a multipayer system with authority
and control dispersed among a thousand sickness
funds that negotiate payment rates with hospitals and
physician associations. Government's direct role in
financing and administering the system is actually
smaller than in the United States. It establishes the
rules, however, and sanctions private bodies to per-
form these functions in pursuit of agreed-on goals.
The process is unique among industrialized nations,
growing out of a social consensus dating back to
Bismarck.

The famous chancellor created the rudiments of
the modern health care system in 1883 with a law that
provided cash payments and direct medical services
to industrial workers who became sick. Together with

a law providing old-age pensions, this became the basis of today's larger social insurance system. A principle of social "solidarity" ensures that everyone enjoys a certain level of well-being, including freedom from the financial risk of serious illness. This principle serves as bedrock for the social insurance systems of other Western European nations as well. Only Germany, however, uses quasi-public entities to enforce it in health care.

Financing and Coverage

Nine of ten Germans are enrolled in statutory sickness funds, which economist Uwe Reinhardt likens to Blue Cross and Blue Shield plans in the United States and which he considers "private socialism" at its best.[1] The funds are organized by region, craft, or company. Blue-collar workers have no real choice of funds, but white-collar workers can choose from several nationwide *Ersatzkassen*, or substitute funds. The benefit packages offered by the funds are tightly regulated by federal law and quite uniform (and comprehensive). But the cost to members is not so uniform, giving the white-collar workers incentives to shop around.

The funds are empowered by the federal government to collect a payroll tax from each member's employer. The total revenue going to each fund pays the costs of covered benefits for all members of the fund. The actuarial health risks of enrollees vary, however, so that tax rates vary among funds; they range widely from a low of about 8 percent up to a

---

1. Kris Kyes, "Health Care in Germany—A Conversation with Uwe E. Reinhardt, Ph.D.," *Decisions in Imaging Economics*, vol. 5, no. 2 (Spring 1992), pp. 18–23.

high of 16 percent, with the average just under 13 percent. The German system spreads risk—and cost—among defined groups of workers rather than across the general population through general taxation. In this regard, it looks much more like the United States, where employee groups are experience-rated, than like Canada, where contributions are uniform across a province.

Because workers pay half the contribution, these differentials in contribution rates undermine the principle of social solidarity, especially since white-collar workers can seek out substitute funds with lower rates—in effect resulting in risk selection. This substitution is causing dissatisfaction among workers and creating pressure for interfund transfers to reduce the differentials and maintain the kind of cross-subsidization that the broad social insurance model implies.

Germany has a private insurance market, which, though much smaller than in the United States, is more significant than in other European countries. The 10 percent of Germans who are privately insured include the self-employed, civil servants who do not participate in sickness funds, and higher-paid workers who are allowed to opt out of those funds. Some sickness fund members also purchase supplementary coverage in the private market, thereby gaining access to private hospital rooms and the personal services of senior physicians—neither of which is provided by the statutory benefit package.

Any German whose income is above a statutory threshold (which is tied to national changes in annual wages and currently is about $35,000) can opt out of the sickness funds. Only about a third of those eligible actually do purchase private coverage, either to gain access to the superior inpatient services or to enjoy premiums that are below the funds' contribution rates. The private insurers' share of the market has grown a little in the past few years, but continued rapid growth is unlikely for political reasons: it would be seen as a threat to the solidarity principle that underlies Germany's entire social insurance system.

Administration and Spending Control

If Germany's decentralized, multipayer system of employment-based sickness funds looks like familiar terrain to Americans, the ground rules for administering this system are uniquely German. The informal corporatist model of publicly sanctioned private negotiations, with the government serving as the umpire, produces results, because the actors understand their roles and can speak their lines without a script. It all unfolds as an expression of what is called *Konzertierte Aktion*, or concerted action, which is also the name of a national council that meets annually to set broad guidelines for negotiations at the state level. The federal minister of health is the chairman of this council of all the stakeholders; the council also has its own staff of policy experts.

Unlike Canada, the German system does not have a formal global budget for health care, a point that many American analysts tend to overlook. The guidelines developed by the *Konzertierte Aktion* are just that, guidelines. While they are not binding, they do have moral authority with the principal actors in the system, which gives them a legitimacy that politically imposed global budgets may lack. Negotiations then take place at the state level, where associations of sickness funds agree with physicians on binding fee schedules and with hospitals on operating budgets and per diem payment rates derived from them.

The guidelines produced from such concerted action have the implicit goal of keeping total spending on health care from growing any faster than the nation's gross national product. A recent report from the council's own panel of experts, however, voices doubts that Germany can keep up with the pace of medical progress while keeping the health care sector from growing as a share of the national economy or GNP.[2] This report is stirring controversy.

As an exception to the general rule, formal global budgets have been in place since 1985 for the payment of outpatient care physicians (inpatient care is delivered by salaried hospital staff physicians, and paid for as part of hospital per diem rates). Outpatient services account for about 20 percent of total spending. The budget caps were established as a "temporary" measure when major changes were made in the relative value scale used to price these services because of uncertainty about how the changes would affect utilization. The effectiveness of the caps in constraining the growth of spending on outpatient care, though, has made the sickness funds reluctant to abandon them.

Not surprisingly, physicians have grown restive under the caps and are seeking their removal. The cap limits the rate of increase in spending for outpatient physician services to the rate of increase in economywide wage levels. The sickness funds give the negotiated capitation to the state physicians' association, which distributes it to individual doctors on a fee-for-service basis according to the relative value

2. Ibid., pp. 20–21.

scale. This is a zero-sum game; if utilization increases too much, fees are automatically reduced to keep total spending under the cap—which is exactly what has been happening in a country where utilization review is minimal compared with the United States.

In effect, each physician's income depends partly on the behavior of other physicians. This works nicely in a staff-model health maintenance organization like Kaiser or a multispecialty group practice like the Mayo Clinic in the United States, where doctors share the same incentives. But German physicians remain individual practitioners and do not appreciate having their incomes depend on the style of medical practice of other practitioners. In addition, Germany is suffering from a veritable glut of physicians, which contributes further to increasing utilization and declining fees.

Until now, Germany has unquestionably been the most successful of Western nations at limiting the rate of increase in total health care spending. Critics of the American system like to use spending as a share of GNP to show how badly we do compared with all other industrialized countries. But this is a seriously flawed measure because of the variability in the rates of GNP growth among nations and over time. By the best measure for comparative purposes, spending per capita, the United States is not such an "outlier" in controlling spending. Indeed, our record is not much different from Canada's over the past decade. But Germany's record is much better than either country's (figure 3–1). Indeed, the only industrialized country that has been as successful at containing spending is Japan, another society with a unique set of quasi-public mechanisms based on a broad social consensus.

FIGURE 3–1
Index of Real (Inflation-adjusted) per Capita National Health Expenditures in Germany, the United States, and Canada, 1970–1990
(1975 = 1.00)

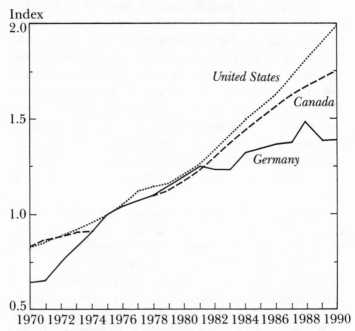

Source: Organization for Economic Cooperation and Development, *The OECD Health Data Program*, software package, English version, 1991.

Reasons for Germany's Success

It is not easy to identify the reasons for Germany's success in limiting the growth of spending on health care. Coverage is comprehensive and virtually universal, while copayments and deductibles are small by American standards. There are no obvious queues of people waiting for nonemergency services, as in Britain and Canada. And there is none of the rigorous review by third parties to control utilization, which is unique to our system.

What, then, are the reasons? To start, cost containment is an explicit goal of government policy, set forth in the Cost Containment Act of 1977. The stated objective is to keep the growth of health care spending in line with that of wages and salaries—without limiting access to necessary care. The *Konzertierte Aktion* was created by this law to serve as the means of guiding all the stakeholders in the system toward that objective; in Germany's culture of social consensus, this seems to have worked.

Germany has more physicians and hospital beds per capita than the United States and higher utilization of both inpatient and outpatient services. Whereas we try to control spending by controlling utilization, the Germans rely more on price controls. But these are not the result of government edict, as in our own Medicare program. Rather, they result from bargaining between private payers and providers over fixed budgets for individual hospitals and for outpatient physicians as a group.

German hospitals may provide more days of care, but they do so with less intensive use of medical resources than do U.S. hospitals. They employ only about a third as many staff per occupied bed (1.53 versus 5.16 in 1988, according to the American Hospital Association and the Deutsche Krankenhausgesellschaft).[3] They also use less capital equipment and have seriously limited investment in new hospital cap-

---

3. Elliot K. Wicks, *German Health Care: Financing, Administration and Coverage* (Washington, D.C.: Health Insurance Association of America, 1992), p. 18.

FIGURE 3–2
Availability of Selected Medical Technologies
in Germany and the United States, 1987

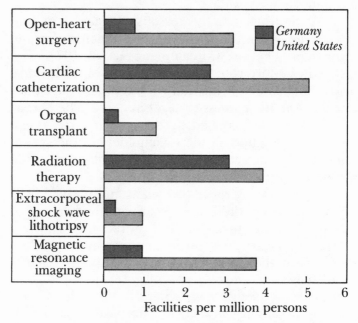

Facilities per million persons

NOTE: Data for German open-heart surgery facilities and organ transplantation facilities are for 1988.
SOURCE: Dale A. Rublee, "Medical Technology in Canada, Germany, and the United States," *Health Affairs*, vol. 8, no. 3 (Fall 1989).

ital, which declined nearly one-fifth in real terms during the 1980s. Certain expensive technologies also are more limited, especially open-heart surgery units and magnetic resonance imaging devices (figure 3–2).

Acquisition of high-technology equipment is the one area of health care spending that is controlled directly by the government in Germany. All hospital capital expenditures are financed through state budgets, while operating costs are covered by the sickness funds. These capital allocations from the states result from a regional planning process similar to the largely ineffective certificate-of-need process in the United States. In Germany, however, the process has been effective in controlling the growth of capital.

Germans visit the doctor more often than Americans, but the nation still spends less on outpatient physician care. Part of the reason lies in the caps placed on payments to ambulatory care physicians in 1985, which have reduced these physicians' incomes relative to those of German workers in general. Doctors' incomes were 4.3 times the compensation of all private sector employees in 1985; by 1989, this figure had fallen to 4.0 times (according to data from Simone Sandier at CREDES in Paris, and from the Organization for Economic Cooperation and Development).[4] German physicians are paid relatively less than their American counterparts, who earned 5.6 times the average compensation for all private sector workers in the United States in 1989.[5] Moreover, the ratio has been running the other way here, with doctors' incomes increasing relative to those of workers in general.

Germans spend much more of their health care dollar (or mark) on drugs than we do, even in absolute terms. Per capita spending for drugs in 1988 was $198 there, compared with $170 here, and accounted for 17 percent of total health care expenditures (only 8 percent here). This situation led to a 1989 law that

4. Ibid., p. 53.
5. Ibid.

reduces payment to the cost of the least expensive generic drug in a class determined to be therapeutically equivalent. As a result, drug companies have reduced their prices dramatically, apparently convinced that Germans would not make large copayments and therefore would choose the least costly drug in a class.

Germany's Problems and Prospects

Despite its apparent success in containing the growth of spending, the German health care system faces some challenges. The report of its own policy experts questioning whether Germany could continue to keep spending from rising any faster than national income—without denying people access to all the fruits of medical progress—was a warning shot across the bow of all national health systems. All these countries are facing the same upward pressures on costs and spending, and must deal with them in one way or another.

Strange as it may sound, health care experts in Germany regularly cite the inability to control costs as the system's biggest problem. They are particularly concerned that spending is rising faster than wages, a situation that, in a system financed entirely by payroll taxes, raises the same kind of issue concerning intergenerational equity that social security raises in the United States. Not surprisingly, it is raising concerns about Germany's international competitiveness as well. These experts also complain that Germans lack incentives to be cost-conscious in their use of health care and so overutilize the system—aided and abetted by the surplus of physicians inducing demand for their services. These complaints could be coming from American policy analysts.

There also is concern that the principle of social solidarity is starting to erode. Although Germans do not like to use the term, risk selection is going on among some of the sickness funds, as higher-income workers choose the substitute funds. While this would hardly be startling news in the United States, it runs counter to the entire philosophy on which the larger German system of social insurance is founded. That system depends on the willingness of the young to subsidize the old and of higher-income citizens to subsidize those of lesser means. In a country with a population older than ours and aging even more rapidly, any breakdown in this long-standing social consensus must be viewed with alarm.

The situation is complicated further by the recent incorporation of East Germany, which one Wall Street analyst called the "biggest leveraged buyout in history." The situation is the rough equivalent of our incorporating Mexico with its health care system. The cost of bringing eastern German health care up to the standard of the rest of the country could be enormous, although the per capita increase in costs is alleviated by adding 17 million to the per capita count.

The most serious threat to spending control may be the likelihood that physicians, watching their relative incomes decline for seven years, will force the cap off expenditures for ambulatory care. Tentative agreements already have been reached with some sickness funds to do just this. If all the funds agreed, the forces pushing in the other direction—an aging population and an oversupply of doctors—would make it hard to keep spending for physician services from rising much faster.

German physicians are accustomed to practicing almost as they please. Unlike their American counterparts, they accepted price controls to retain their clinical freedom from outside review. They show no interest in the managed-care approach that is emerging as our strategy for improving the cost-effectiveness of the health care system. Indeed, the Dutch and even the British are far ahead of them in starting to adopt some of the elements of managed care to control costs.

More nations are gradually accepting the idea that holding providers accountable for their performance is one of the keys to controlling *costs* generated within the system. Price controls, still Germany's strategy of choice, merely try to control total *spending* by the system. With these controls breaking down for physicians, Germany may have no choice but to try a new approach aimed at better managing the utilization of services.

Lessons for the United States

In returning to the question of whether Germany is now *the* model for the United States, a famous statement of Bismarck's comes to mind: "The less people know about how laws and sausages are made, the better." Germany's health care system is an elaborate sausage, with a mixture of ingredients designed for, and palatable to, German tastes and traditions. Because American tastes and traditions are different, transplanting anything as complex and subtle as the German system to these shores is difficult to imagine. It is the product of a different history and the expression of a different philosophy, difficult to describe to outsiders.

Conceivably, certain features of the German system could be adapted to the American setting, such as its unique design for ensuring universal coverage while maintaining decentralized administration. In this sense, it is a more appropriate model than the monolithic Canadian single-payer system derived from the British model. Germany will soon find itself having to adopt some American ideas about managed care, however, to slow the increase in utilization that jeopardizes its ability to control total spending. Indeed, the health care systems of all nations will be converging to a degree, as the United States provides universal coverage like that of other countries and as the other nations realize the need to improve the performance of the health care sector through application of managed-care principles.

There will be no German-American—or Canadian-American—health care system because the United States is neither Germany nor Canada. No country is a model for any other, but all must resolve the same fundamental dilemma: how to ensure aging populations access to the useful fruits of medical progress without breaking the bank. In this undertaking, all can learn from one another.

FOUR

Lessons from the Netherlands

Warren Greenberg

The most important lesson one can learn from the Netherlands is that a deregulated health care system can be devised to let managed-care plans be managed-care plans for all Americans, including those who are currently uninsured or underinsured, rather than cream-skimming plans that deny coverage to high-risk individuals. Public policy, therefore, should create incentives for managed-care plans to contain costs and should curb incentives to avoid individuals who most need health insurance.

A second lesson is that a regulated health care system not only may be inefficient but need not guarantee equity in coverage. In contrast, a movement to a more competitive system can be compatible with efficiency as well as increases in the equity of coverage.

First, I discuss the current highly regulated health care system in the Netherlands and the frustrations of this cartelized system. Second, I describe the proposed health care system in the Netherlands, which has been approved by both the Center-Left and the Center-Right political parties. The proposed system relies on competition and managed-care plans with universal coverage. Third, I suggest some lessons from the proposed Dutch health care system to achieve efficiency and equity in the U.S. health care system.

The Current Dutch System

The current health care system in the Netherlands is two-tiered. Individuals who make less than $25,000 a year or who are unemployed must enroll in a sickness fund in their geographic area. Approximately two-thirds of the population are enrolled in such plans.

Physicians who are in medical specialties practice on a fee-for-service basis in the sickness funds. General practitioners are paid on a capitation basis. Hospital rates are negotiated on a per diem basis. Sickness funds have no incentives to operate efficiently, because they are reimbursed by the government on the basis of the health expenditures of their members. Indeed, a sickness fund that improves efficiency sees its revenues decrease.

Physicians are exempt from antitrust laws that would prohibit boycotts of utilization review activities by sickness funds. Physicians may also collude on the price or size of the market that they serve without regard to the antitrust authorities. Selective contracting of hospitals or physicians is not allowed by the sickness funds. Preferred provider organizations are not legal. Utilization review does not exist because of potential boycotts by providers against insuring organizations, and managed care does not exist either.

There are substantial barriers to entry for both physicians and hospitals. Physicians may not practice in particular areas without approval of the physicians already in the area. For-profit hospitals are not allowed. There is substantial regulation of the number of hospital beds and technology in each region of the country. Financing of the sickness funds comes from premiums paid both by the employer and by the employee.

Those in the remaining one-third of the population whose annual incomes are greater than $25,000 or who are self-employed may attempt to enroll with one of the seventy competing commercial insurers. Physicians and hospitals negotiate uniform payments with all commercial insurers. Financing of the commercial insurers is derived from premiums paid by both the employer and the employee. Tactics such as changing the benefit plan design to enroll the lowest-risk individuals is the most prominent form of competition among the commercial insurers.

In summary, the current Dutch health care system is highly cartelized with little consumer choice among sickness funds; choice in the commercial insurance market is limited to the health status of the enrollee. The government plays a conspicuous regulatory role since entry of providers, new technology, and new investment must be approved by the government. Approximately 8.5 percent of the gross national product in the Netherlands went to health care in the early 1990s, compared with 3.3 percent in 1953.

Movement to a New Health Care System

The proposed Dutch health care system is an attempt to combine competition, efficiency, and equity. The proposals grew out of a March 1987 report by the

Committee on the Structure and Financing of Health Care, an advisory committee set up by the Netherlands government; the chairman was the president of the Board of Directors of Phillips Corporation, Wisse Dekker.[1] The Dutch government has been in broad agreement with the recommendations of the Dekker committee, and implementation of new legislation has begun. The proposals are targeted for implementation by 1995, but delays in implementation may be likely.

The new system is based on the consumer-choice health plan first proposed by Stanford University professor Alain Enthoven in the *New England Journal of Medicine* in 1978.[2] Each individual will select a health plan from competing insuring organizations such as PPOs, health maintenance organizations, or indemnity plans during an open-enrollment period every two years. Employers can pay up to one-half of the nominal health care premium for an employee if they desire. The government will require each insuring organization to offer a substantially similar benefit package to prevent skimpy benefit packages from being used to attract only the healthiest persons. The benefit package will cover nearly all acute care, long-term care, and health-related social welfare expenses. Individuals will also be free to purchase a supplemental plan to pay for discretionary cosmetic surgery, abortions, and hospital amenities, such as private rooms, from among competing insuring organiza-

---

1. Committee on the Structure and Financing of Health Care, *Willingness to Change* (The Hague, Netherlands: Distribution Center for Government Publications, March 1987).
2. Alain Enthoven, "Consumer-Choice Health Plan," *New England Journal of Medicine*, vol. 298, nos. 12, 13 (1978), pp. 650–58, 709–20.

tions. Individuals will pay health insurance premiums based proportionately on their income into a central fund. If they desire, employers can contribute to the central fund in addition to the employee. Unemployed individuals will pay only a modest premium.

The central fund, in turn, will reimburse each health-insuring organization based on the mixture of individuals who joined the organization. Organizations that attract mostly chronically ill or elderly individuals will receive a greater reimbursement than those that attract younger populations. By reimbursing insuring organizations on a case-mixture basis, the plan creates incentives to enroll individuals who will incur greater health care expenses. This is the least regulatory of any mechanism that can eliminate cream skimming.

Nevertheless, the computation of the case-mixture reimbursement is a difficult research task. Thus far, researchers have been able to explain approximately two-thirds of the maximum explainable variance of about 15 percent in individual health expenditures with case-mixture measures.[3] Approximately 85 percent of the variance in individual health care expenditures is simply unexplained and unpredictable. Case-mixture measures need not be perfect, however, because insuring organizations will also not be able to forecast their population and their expenses with precision.

Insuring organizations may compete on their ability to contain costs, to be efficient, and to offer quality health care and responsive service to their

---

3. Joseph P. Newhouse, Willard G. Manning, Emmett B. Keeler, and E. H. Sloss, "Adjusting Capitation Rates Using Objective Health Resources and Prior Utilization," *Health Care Financing Review*, vol. 10, no. 3 (1989), pp. 41–54.

subscribers. Insuring organizations may compete on the quality of physicians and hospitals in their preferred provider organization network. Insuring organizations may compete on convenience of location of their providers or the lack of waiting lines. Insuring organizations may also charge an optional premium so that the average of all premiums is 11 percent above the amount paid by the central fund. This additional premium is independent of one's income and can vary by insuring organization, creating incentives for insuring organizations to be efficient so that they can reduce premiums.

There will also be a substantial antitrust component to prevent providers from boycotting cost-containment efforts of the managed-care plans as well as to prevent managed-care plans from colluding on price or segmenting the market. Consumer information on the characteristics, costs, and benefits of each plan will be provided by the insuring organizations, employers, the government, and private consumer protection groups. Health care costs will be controlled by competition among managed-care plans as well as by limits on the use of expensive technology.

Lessons for the United States

First, the Dutch government and people found a heavily regulated health care system to be inefficient and unworkable. Second, competition among health-insuring organizations using managed-care techniques was found to be a desirable alternative. Although there will be less regulation and micromanagement of providers and technology, the government will still have a role in antitrust enforcement, consumer protection, and the setting of case-mixture adjusted reimbursement formulas to constrain cream skimming. Finally, as before, universal health care coverage is the highest priority.

What can the United States learn from the Netherlands to achieve an efficient and equitable health care system? The optimal strategy would be to move away from an almost complete reliance on an employer-based health care system. Employers could still, however, pay health care premiums for employees and provide information on the relative value of the health care plans that an employee might consider. Instead of the employer-based system, individuals could purchase insurance at specified open-enrollment periods whether they are working for a large employer or small employer, are self-employed, are in between jobs, or are unemployed. That is, employment status should not be a determinant of an individual's securing insurance coverage.

To reduce the tendency for competing insuring organizations to avoid high-risk individuals, the insuring organizations must be reimbursed by the government on a case-mixture basis. Regulating the types of individuals that an insuring organization will enroll as well as the premiums will be far more intrusive and ineffectual than reimbursing firms that accept high-risk individuals. Finally, let managed-care plans compete to contain costs without government intervention and control of provider prices and output. If these principles were followed, the uncertainties and inequities of reliance on an employer-based system for health insurance would no longer exist.

The advantages of moving away from an employer-based to an individual-based health insurance system might be summarized as follows. All individuals could purchase a health insurance plan regardless of health or income status. Individuals who lost jobs in a recession would not also lose their health insurance benefits. All individuals would have a choice of a health insurance plan rather than being tied to a single plan offered by their employer. Nearly two-thirds of all employees of medium and large firms in the United States are not offered a choice of plan by their employer.[4]

There would be no productivity loss to the individual or society in the economy because of job lock. Moreover, the duration of unemployment might be reduced if individuals could secure health insurance without being excluded for preexisting conditions. In addition, employers would not have to bear the added costs of reverse job lock. Reverse job lock occurs when individuals who are previously uninsured take a position with a firm that offers health insurance benefits when they become sick. This reverse job lock, or adverse selection, can add substantially to the costs of the new firm. Reverse job lock may lead over time to exclusion clauses for existing conditions by the new firm.

There would be no distortion or excess welfare loss due to premiums paid by employers that are currently not subject to income taxes. This distortion leads individuals to purchase greater amounts of health insurance than would be the case if premiums paid by employers were taxed. This distortion benefits higher-income individuals and leads to the purchase of greater amounts of health insurance.

The high costs of health insurance now borne directly by many employers would no longer add to

4. Gail A. Jensen et al., "Cost Sharing and the Changing Pattern of Employer-sponsored Health Benefits," *Milbank Quarterly*, vol. 65, no. 4 (1987), pp. 521–50.

the price of a firm's product if a firm decided not to pay health insurance premiums. These firms would no longer be put at a competitive disadvantage relative to firms that do not offer health insurance or to foreign firms that do not pay health insurance premiums. (A reduction in health insurance benefits may take the form of increased wages.)

Individuals would no longer lose their health insurance if their employers became bankrupt. Employees enrolled with employers that are self-insured under the Employment Retirement Income Security Act (more than one-third of the work force) would no longer live with the uncertainty about when their health insurance may be terminated. Under the *H&H Music* case, which was recently affirmed by the New Orleans Court of Appeals, employers have the right to terminate or reduce an employee's insurance policy without notice.[5] Unlike play-or-pay proposals, small businesses would not have health insurance requirements imposed on them. Such requirements may eventually lead to increased unemployment.

Intrusive government regulation would not be needed as health-insuring organizations competed on varying dimensions of price and quality. Government planning would not be needed. A case-mixture adjusted reimbursement formula would have to be devised to allow insuring organizations to compete on cost containment and not on avoiding high-risk individuals.[6]

---

5. John McGann v. H&H Music Company no. 90-2672, U.S. Court of Appeals for the Fifth Circuit, 946 F.2d 401. 1991 U.S. App. Lexis 26056.
6. See, for example, James Lubitz, "Health Status Adjustments for Medicare Capitation," *Inquiry*, vol. 24, no. 4 (1984), pp. 362–75; and Wynand P. M. M. van de Ven and Rene C. J. A. Van Vliet, "How Can We Prevent Cream Skimming in a Competitive Health

The United States might gain some lessons from the dissatisfaction of the Dutch with their current regulated system and their desire to move to a more competitive system: the United States should not do away with market forces but, indeed, should make the health care system more competitive and vibrant. At the same time, the Dutch reforms emphasize guaranteeing health insurance coverage for all individuals regardless of their income, health, or employment status. Competition need not be sacrificed as a health system moves toward more equitable coverage, nor should the concern for equity in health care be a reason to limit market forces.

Insurance Market?" in Peter Zweifel and H. E. Frech III, *Health Economics Worldwide* (Dordrecht, Netherlands: Kluwer Academic Publishers, 1992), pp. 23–46.

FIVE

Lessons from the United Kingdom

Alan Maynard

In the twenty-five years I have been visiting the United States and analyzing its health care system, it has become more and more apparent how the problems facing it are similar to those faced by the British national health care system. It is always stimulating to examine both the diversity of U.S. health care systems (for example, Medicare, Medicaid, U.A., Blue Cross and Blue Shield, self-insurers, and private insurers) and the vigorous attempts to contain costs and to pursue other social and economic objectives.

The U.K. National Health Service does not have the American problems of access to care. It does, however, experience many other American problems such as identifying what works in terms of cost-effective therapies, explaining the large variations in practitioner behavior (the U.K. equivalent of John E. Wennberg's Boston and New Haven differences in care),[1] and devising appropriate incentives to ensure

---

1. J. E. Wennberg and A. Gittlesohn, "Small Variations in Health Care Delivery," *Science*, vol. 182 (1973), pp. 1102–8.

that both individuals and institutions pursue efficiency in health care delivery rather than objectives such as personal gain and the expansion of unproven therapies.

Characteristics of NHS

Britain's NHS is financed largely out of general taxation; copayments contribute only 5 percent of total revenues. The belief in America is that the NHS is a socialist and highly regulated system. It is socialist in the sense that it provides free access to care regardless of insurance contributions, income, age, and gender.

The NHS is not socialist in the sense that it is not highly regulated. Since 1948, when the NHS was established, the government has preserved medical autonomy. The delivery of health care is, as a consequence, controlled by doctors who tend to work on an individual basis, managed by no one. Clinical autonomy in the U.K. NHS is far greater than it is in the U.S. health care systems. In the United States, practitioner behavior is managed, perhaps quite correctly, in a way that is highly socialist.

The well-publicized problems of the NHS, such as queues and long waits for non-emergency elective procedures and the alleged underuse of high-technology interventions, aroused Mrs. Thatcher when she came into office in 1979. She commissioned a report from a Whitehall think tank, the Central Policy Review Unit. This rather naive report was completed in 1982 and offered the option of the privatization of the U.K. health care system, that is, a move toward an insurance-based health care system with services supplied by private institutions.

The public, academic, and professional reaction

to this report was hostile. Mrs. Thatcher recognized that it was difficult to change the NHS. Approaching the 1983 election, she adopted a pragmatic approach, saying at the Conservative party annual conference in 1982, "The principle that adequate health care should be provided for all, regardless of their ability to pay, must be the foundation for any arrangements for financing health care." Such sentiments have more in common with her socialist predecessors than with the arguments of her apparent gurus, Friedrich Hayek and Milton Friedman.

The "ideal" NHS would deploy resources from its finite budget to those patients who could benefit most from health care. Unfortunately, the level of ignorance is such in all health care systems that re-source allocators, be they managers or clinicians, can-not identify, let alone deliver to patients, interven-tions that are cost-effective.

There was a gradual realization of this deficiency in government. This, together with Mrs. Thatcher's desire to reduce public expenditure (a desire trans-lated into *increased* public expenditure over the 1980s), led to parsimonious funding of the NHS in the 1980s.

Tight expenditure controls led to crises in the provision of health care in 1987, with the media identifying spectacular cases of patients' failing to get treatment and being left to die. Mrs. Thatcher re-sponded by instigating a review of the NHS. This was carried out in secret, without sunshine laws like those in the United States; the precise nature of these deliberations will not be known for thirty years.

What problems were discussed in public during this review? It was publicly recognized, after thirty years, that the NHS operates with insufficient data and with little management. The costs of treatments are unknown: there are no prices to give even a ballpark figure of the consequences on resources of a practitioner's decision to repair, for instance, a hernia. The managers of NHS hospitals have no patient or activity data to inform their choices: typically, they do not know what their doctors are doing or how many patients are in the hospital at any one time.

The Thatcher government's decision to challenge the NHS and clinicians about this issue destroyed a consensus that had existed since 1948: the medical profession determined and was not questioned by the political process about who got what services, while the state decided the level of public expenditure on the NHS. Mrs. Thatcher would not tolerate the maintenance of clinical autonomy: in the future, medical practitioners were to be accountable. She decided in the popular jargon of the 1980s to "handbag" the physicians and surgeons. This verb, recognized internationally by George Shultz when he retired as U.S. secretary of state and presented Mrs. Thatcher with a handbag, describes nicely the vigor of her response to restrictive practices.

The reforms that emerged in 1989 reflected the advocacy of Alain Enthoven and some of his U.K counterparts who advised the Thatcher government directly and indirectly. There has been a separation of provider and purchaser functions with the creation of contracts to regulate transactions between the two. The purpose of these reforms was to create greater openness and accountability.

Efficiency

For the market to function efficiently, it requires information and efficiency-enhancing rules. Information about costs, activities, and outcomes are essential for efficient trading. Unlike the U.S. system, the U.K. NHS has no price data and poor activity data. Both systems have poor outcome data. A joke in the United Kingdom is that in any hospital it is impossible to distinguish, in existing information bases, between vertical (walking) and horizontal (dead) discharges.

Yet the problem of outcome measurement is old. Frances Clifton, the physician of the Prince of Wales, in *The State of Physic* (1732) argued:

> In order, therefore to procure this valuable collection, I humbly propose, first of all, that three or four persons should be employed in the hospitals (and that without any ways interfering with the gentlemen now concerned), to set down the cases of the patients there from day to day, candidly and judiciously, without any regard to private opinions or public systems, and at the year's end publish these facts just as they are, leaving every one to make the best use he can for himself.[2]

"The gentlemen now concerned" (the clinicians) objected to data collection more than 250 years ago. In the late 1980s, the U.S. government followed Clifton's advice by collecting and publishing hospital mortality records on a regular basis. The U.K. NHS has yet to adopt this ancient advice. Yet without such outcome data, how can purchaser-provider contracts be devised efficiently?

The other important issue in the competitive health care debate is the determination of the rules that affect trading. The Thatcher reforms have been

2. Quoted in editorial, *Lancet*, 1841, pp. 650–51.

developed in an increasingly restrictive manner. The administration has been fearful, particularly in the 1992 campaign, of the effects of competition. As a result, it subsidized marginal London suppliers and, by doing so, avoided hospital closures. It also fixed the maximum rate of return on capital, thus constraining price competition. The clear risk is that, instead of competition, the NHS reform will create a state bureaucracy similar to that removed by Mikhail Gorbachev in the Soviet Union.

What will be the outcome of Thatcher reforms of the NHS? The optimistic scenario is that the existing deficits in information (particularly about prices and outcomes) will be reduced and management will be better informed in identifying what is cost-effective in the morass of unproven health care interventions. The pessimistic scenario is that clinical autonomy will be eroded and replaced by an expensive, rigid, and ill-informed bureaucracy.

What are the lessons for the United States? Regarding access, public finance is a useful tool both to increase equity and to gain control over cost inflations (by the single pipe of funding). The common U.S.-U.K. issue of efficiency in the supply of health care requires careful use of the limited knowledge base and a rapid expansion of the investigation of outcomes and cost-effectiveness. The processes both of determining what works and of persuading practitioners to abandon the unproven and adopt the cost-effective will provide opportunities for much mutual learning between the U.S. and the U.K. practitioner, between the policy and the research communities.

The political problem common to all health care systems is that those in government tend to respond to poorly defined, often media-induced "crises" with unproven and risky reform policies. This creates the risk of much turmoil and change in the finance and delivery of health care but all too little improvement in the efficiency and access of the health care system. This problem is not new, as Caius Petronius, an administrator who worked for the Roman Emperor Nero, remarked:

> We trained very hard, but it seemed that every time we were beginning to form up into teams, we would be reorganized. I was to learn later in life that we tend to meet any new situation by reorganizing, and a wonderful method it can be for creating the illusion of progress, while producing confusion, inefficiency, and demoralization.

A Note on the Book

This book was edited by Ann Petty and Dana Lane of the
publications staff of the American Enterprise Institute.
The figures were drawn by Hördur Karlsson.
The text was set in Baskerville.
Coghill Composition Company of Richmond, Virginia,
set the type, and Edwards Brothers Incorporated,
of Ann Arbor, Michigan, printed and bound the book,
using permanent acid-free paper.

The AEI Press is the publisher for the American Enterprise
Institute for Public Policy Research, 1150 17th Street, N.W.,
Washington, D.C. 20036; *Christopher C. DeMuth,* publisher; *Edward*
Styles, director; *Dana Lane,* assistant director; *Ann Petty,* editor;
Cheryl Weissman, editor; *Mary Cristina Delaney,* editorial assistant
(rights and permissions).